Is There a Cure for Cancer

Natural Alternative Cancer Treatments

David Gaughan

Is There a Cure for Cancer

Natural Alternative Cancer Treatments

The treatments, foods and diet listed here is for information only. They are not recommendations for or against any other treatments or therapies. The decision of whether to have traditional medical treatment, alternative treatment or a combination of both is up to each individual to decide for themselves.

.

Preface

Is there a cure for cancer? This question has plagued humanity throughout the ages and particularly over the past century where incidences of cancer have ballooned. And yet, the cure for cancer may be simply what we put in our mouths. In our modern age of fast food convenience and little time, we've lost the knowledge of what certain foods provide for essential health.

Many experts believe that cancer is in all of us, but it is only when our immune systems are depleted that the disease takes over. If you give the body what it needs with a program of natural remedies and cancer diet therapy, it will surprise you with how quickly it responds, even with chronic illness.

So how does the body heal itself? It heals through a strengthened immune system. As we age, the immune system weakens. When we give it a boost, it fights its own battles, finding its own cure or remedy for multiple illnesses, including cancer.

The majority of these natural remedies and treatments involve pure substances that are popular around the world. The information is available on the internet, although often with an overload of information to wade through to get to the most important material. It has been simplified here to save you research time, giving you the condensed information of the most commonly used natural remedies to help the body heal itself.

Boosting the immune system helps the body find its own cure with its stronger immune system. The alternative treatments, foods and diet listed here provide a program to help the body heal itself. They are not recommendations for or against any other treatments or therapies. Readers are encouraged to do further research to clarify any queries regarding these natural immune system support remedies. The decision of whether to have traditional medical treatment, alternative treatment or a combination of both is up to each individual to decide for themselves.

List of Contents:

Overview of Cancer Treatment Essentials

Every body produces cancer cells, but the cancer only takes over when the body is depleted and unable to fight. Any cancer treatment must include four essential elements:

I. **Strengthen the immune system**: a healthy immune system will kill cancer cells faster than the body can produce them.

II. **Oxygenate the cells**: cancer thrives on sugar and struggles in a highly oxygenated system.

III. **Detoxify the body**: the immune system struggles with heavy metal toxins and our modern life loads us with toxins daily. The body copes up to a point, but a detox program will help give the immune system a boost.

IV. **Change the body chemistry from acidic to alkaline**: our modern diet and lifestyle tends to make our bodies acidic and cancer thrives in acidic systems. When you change your body chemistry to alkaline, particularly through diet, you give your body a fighting chance. A vegetarian diet with no dairy is recommended by many. One reason to eliminate dairy is because it is highly acidic. The one exception is cottage cheese when used in combination with flax seed oil, as noted later in this package.

When determining a treatment for cancer, conventional or otherwise, consider whether the treatment incorporates the above four essentials.

Basic Preliminaries:

Help Your Body Find its Own Cure

A. Cut down on sugar intake (and carbohydrates):

Low sugar Diets seem to starve cancer cells. Research shows that cancer cells seem to use sugar as their basic "fuel". Increased sugar intake seems to increase body conditions that encourage cancer to grow. Ideally, your main sugar intake would be from fruit. Maple syrup can be a better substitute for sugar than artificial sweeteners, but keep it to a minimum – see upcoming heading for Baking soda, combined with Maple Syrup for targeting tumor growths (#5 in the "Simple Low-Cost Treatments" section).

Damaged cancerous cells are able to thrive and replicate as long as the person provides them with an abundant supply of glucose. People who eat a carbohydrate-rich diet are making themselves fertile ground for cancer. If you deny them glucose, it's a challenge for cancer cells to stay alive. Those that do survive can most likely be eliminated by your immune system.

Toronto researchers found that microbes in your intestine convert carbohydrates into metabolites that spur cancer growth. A low-carbohydrate diet shut down this process and led to a whopping 75 per cent reduction in cancer incidence in their animal study!

if you have cancer it's imperative to stop eating all sugar, in any form, as well as refined carbohydrates like flour and other high-glycemic foods like potatoes and rice. You can thereby starve cancer cells of glucose, the food they need to live.

B. Increase Water intake:

The majority of people are under hydrated, drinking beverages that are diuretics rather than clean water. Water is one of the most essential elements of good health. It maintains system equilibrium, lubricates, flushes wastes and toxins, hydrates the skin, regulates body temperature, adds needed minerals and transports nutrients, minerals, vitamins, proteins etc. The human body is predominantly water, so without water the body can survive only a few days. The body can store water, but only on a very limited basis. The average person should consume 8 to 10 eight ounce glasses of water each day.

C. Detox:

Many health practitioners recommend detoxing the body before treatment – they consider it an essential part of treatment. Effective ways to detoxify the body include liver flush, colon cleansing, fasting, chelation.

There are also detoxification aids in the form of nutritional, herbal and homeopathic remedies and some people prefer the more gentle detoxing methods. One simple one is the **brown rice diet**, where only whole grain brown rice is eaten for several days, chewing each mouthful 30 to 100 times to get the full nutritional benefit and to detox the body. Also, a 100% plant and whole food diet has a natural detoxing effect.

Another simple method for detoxing the body and improving health, particularly oral health is **Coconut oil Pulling**, where coconut oil (or any other vegetable oil) is swilled in the mouth for up to twenty minutes and then expelled. This draws out toxins through the tongue and mouth with reportedly great health results. We've included a separate section on oil pulling later, but you can do an internet search on *Coconut oil Pulling* for additional details.

Some health practitioners recommend the full liver flush as noted below, especially for people with advanced illness. They also recommend an enema to flush excess waste and toxins from the body, although this option is not to everyone's preference – if you prefer not to include the enema, ensure you take extra roughage, maybe in the form of psyllium husks to absorb toxins and pass them quickly through the bowels to minimize the risk of re-absorption into the body.

For those choosing the enema option, introducing coffee into the enema supposedly causes the liver to release stored up toxins into the digestive system to be eliminated.

D. Liver Flush:

A simple liver flush involves Epsom salts, followed by a mix of olive oil and grapefruit juice (or lemon juice). This might be a bit harsh for some people, particularly those who have an adverse reaction to the Epsom salts. A milder form of liver flush is noted below, but many health practitioners recommend the full liver flush as per Dr. Hulda Clark 's method.

Dr. Hulda Clark recommended a parasite cleanse first because you can't clean a liver with live parasites. Use a zapper for one week prior to the liver cleanse or, if you don't have access to a zapper, drink a herbal tea morning and night of wormwood, cloves and black walnut. Preferably make tea from dried herbs if available from the health store or Chinese supply store. Alternatively, many health stores have parasite cleanse and liver flush tinctures or homeopathic remedies that will achieve the same result.

Some health practitioners also recommend drinking apple juice for several days prior to the flush – this helps soften stones. Do a search on Dr. Hulda Clark liver flush for full details.

On the morning of the liver flush start with a light, no-fat breakfast and lunch – do not eat or drink after two pm. Mix 4 tablespoons of Epsom Salts in 3 cups water and pour this into a jar – if preferred, refrigerate for taste. This makes four servings, 3/4 (three fourths) cup each time. At 6.00pm drink one serving 3/4 (three fourths cup) of the Epsom salts mix. At 8.00pm repeat by drinking another 3/4 (three fourths) cup of Epsom salts mix. Pour half cup (measured) olive oil into a jar and mix with freshly squeezed juice (3 lemons or 1 large grapefruit to make ¾ cup of juice). The grapefruit juice mixes best. Screw lid on jar and shake well to mix. Let sit for about fifteen minutes, then shake again. The lemon juice can transform the oil into a gel-like consistency, so some people might prefer to sip alternately from the oil and lemon juice until finished. At 10.00 pm, drink the potion you have mixed. Preferably drink it in sips – or through a large straw. Next morning, upon awakening take your third dose of Epsom salts, after 6.00am. Two hours later take your fourth (the last) dose of Epsom salts.

Note: Do a search on Dr. Hulda Clark liver flush for full details.

Milder Liver Flush:

For those who find the above a bit grueling, a milder form was prescribed by Edgar Cayce, the famous American "Sleeping Prophet". Cayce prescribed a three-day apple diet where for three days you eat nothing but apples, preferably organic types like Jonathans, Delicious, Oregon reds, Arkansas black, plus water. At the end of the third day, two tablespoons of olive oil is taken.

Increasing your water intake, as noted previously, may be one of the best ways to get rid of toxins in the body, particularly after a detoxification program.

E. Diet & Nutrition:

Health professionals often suggest, particularly for cancer cases, increasing fresh vegetables and fruit intake, plus avoidance of animal fats. Again, the famous Edgar Cayce who, while in a trancelike hypnotic state, often prescribed treatments for medical conditions. He suggested the fruit and vegetable diet is preferable, with no processed foods. The fats should be more from nuts rather than meats, especially cashew nuts, almonds, filberts (hazelnuts) etc. He particularly recommended Almonds.

Okay, the above are the basics, but there's another thing to Consider

F. Remove Root Canals

Might sound strange, but there are many who believe that oral hygiene plays a big part in damaging the immune system. Root canals in particular have been linked to many health problems, including cancer. Root canals are prone to inflammation, causing pockets of toxins in the jaw that circulate back into the bloodstream on an ongoing basis. This depletes the immune system and a strong immune system is the number one key to fighting cancer.

This is obviously a very controversial subject and you need to do your own research before deciding whether to remove root canals or not.

The #1 Miracle Food for Health

- GREEN SMOOTHIES

If you do nothing else – DO THIS! Add a Green Smoothie to your daily routine.

Green smoothies are the easiest way to "drink" large quantities of fruits and vegetables you wouldn't be able to consume otherwise. It's quick, convenient and, when added to your daily routine, can give your immune system the boost it needs to fight most disease, particularly with the key ingredient listed below.

We're talking about smoothies here, not juicing – it's important to include the whole vegetable and fruit roughage, not just the juice. Smoothies flood your body with plant-based **phytonutrients**, which deliver a wealth of benefits, including a rich source of beneficial amino acids, minerals and antioxidants.

Often described as the "3-Minute Wellness in a Glass" (the time it takes to prepare), a **single green smoothie can fill your nutritional quota** for the day and keep chronic diseases away. This is particularly so with the higher quality organic vegetables and fruits. Depending on your location and financial restraints, if organic is not an option for you, use whatever greens and fruits available, but do try to get organic if possible.

A secret ingredient for enhancing the absorption of nutrients from your green smoothie is to add a little fermented vegetables in the mix, such as sauerkraut – this is covered in more detail in the companion book *Wisdom Wellness Diet – Returning to Health.*

Essentially, the "green smoothie" consists of 60% fruits (fresh or frozen) and 40% green vegetables, blended in a high-powered blender with a cup of liquid. Organic fruits and vegetables are best, but if they're not easily available then use what you can get – the emphasis is on regular consumption of this health tonic. The liquid can be filtered water or a little wheat grass juice, or Rejuvelac if possible. Rejuvelac is a home-made fermented beverage made from soaking grain sprouts in filtered water – more on this is covered in the *Wisdom Wellness Diet – Returning to Health*).

Many health experts maintain that **including just 3 to 4 fruits and at least 3 vegetables in your daily diet gives your body what it needs to fight most disease.** A daily green smoothie is an easy and delicious way to achieve this.

Boost your Immune System – add these foods to your diet

Boosting the immune system is essential for fighting cancer. If the body's defense system is strong, cancer cannot take hold. Many health practitioners believe that boosting the immune system is so important that supplementation is needed for quick results. There are also natural foods that help boost the body's immune system and these should be added to the diet on a regular basis. The main ones are garlic, ginger, Bell peppers and the Indian spice turmeric.

Garlic: Considered a gift from the gods in ancient times, it has virus-fighting and bacteria-killing properties. Add it regularly to your meals. See later section for more information on this wondrous food.

Ginger: this is a natural anti-inflammatory that has been shown to reduce blood clots and cholesterol.

Turmeric: a spice that helps with digestive problems, turmeric contains curcumin, which has antioxidant properties. Turmeric is antibacterial and anti-inflammatory and also has strong cancer-fighting properties as noted later.

Bell peppers: This pepper variety is sweet and crunchy and contains the carotenoid lycopene which lowers the risk of cancer.

Diet – Greens and Enzymes: For people with cancer, greens and enzymes are essential. If you're serious about obtaining and maintaining long-term health, then besides adding the above foods to your diet, you'll consider changing your diet altogether. Many health practitioners recommend a 100% plant based whole foods diet, eliminating sugars, all processed foods, gluten (which converts to glucose and feeds the cancer), plus all animal proteins and dairy products (which are hard to digest and diverts the body energy from fighting cancer). The *Wisdom Wellness Diet* goes into this in detail – find it on the following link http://www.amazon.com/dp/B00B0K1OIG.

Simple Low-Cost Treatments

1. Bicarbonate Maple Syrup Cancer Treatment –

This treatment has been likened to a natural chemotherapy that effectively kills cancer cells but with minimal side effects. It takes advantage of the effect of sugar on cancer cells, where the cancer feeds on the syrup, but in this case it's a delivery system for the baking soda, which kills the cancer cells before they have a chance to grow.

With pure, 100% maple syrup, mixed to baking soda with heat, the substances bind together. Cancer cells, which consume fifteen times more glucose than normal cells, readily absorb the maple syrup along with the baking soda which, being alkaline, changes the pH and kills the cell.

This treatment was reportedly discovered around the middle of last century by Jim Kelmun, a folk healer who was treating a family of five sisters, four of whom had died of breast cancer. When he asked the surviving sister about anything in her diet that was different to her sisters, she mentioned that she was partial to sipping Maple syrup and baking soda.

Mix and Dose Instructions: Add one part baking soda to three parts pure maple syrup and stir briskly in a small saucepan (non-aluminum pan). Mix and stir on low heat for five to ten minutes. Take one teaspoon daily, building up to two or maximum three teaspoons, with minimum two hours between doses. Do not exceed three teaspoons daily.

Ensure your baking soda is aluminum free – plain baking soda only. You can mix a batch to last a maximum nine days and store at room temperature without refrigeration to ensure the mix doesn't separate over time.

This treatment has had reportedly good results for all types of cancer and an even better success rate when used in combination with other safe and effective treatments. Baking soda has been likened to cyanide to cancer cells and allows more oxygen into the cancer cells than they can tolerate.

2. **The Budwig Flax Oil & Cottage Cheese diet**:

Although eliminating dairy in the diet is recommended, cottage cheese is the one exception because this combination of products has been one of the most popular and successful alternative cancer therapies for decades. Apparently when you mix cottage cheese with flax oil it loses its dairy properties. The unique substance seems to kill cancer cells and at the same time makes every other cell in your body healthier.

Scientists believe flaxseed may pack a powerful punch to knock out estrogen-dependent cancers **including breast and prostate cancer**.

After three decades of research Dr. Johanna Budwig, a German biochemist who was nominated for the Nobel Award six-times, found that her simple formula of two tablespoons of flaxseed oil mixed with a quarter cup of low fat cottage cheese (or other foods containing sulfur) helps increase metabolism, boosts the immune system, reduces cholesterol levels and helps inhibit cancer-cell growth. The two products need to be mixed and taken together to work effectively, so it's best to blend in a mixer for best results. Some people choose to add fruit or nuts and take the mix as a meal.

Those on a vegan diet might try substituting the cottage cheese for other sulfur foods, such as almonds or dried apricots. Also, whole-foods proponents recommend taking freshly ground linseed rather than processed oil that is devoid of fiber and can turn rancid after a period of time. However, the original Budwig diet was cottage cheese and flax oil, so it's best to stay with the original formula.

Dr. Budwig holds a Ph.D. in Natural Science, has undergone medical training and was schooled in pharmaceutical science, physics, botany and biology. Her research showed that the blood of seriously ill cancer patients was always deficient in certain important essential ingredients, including phosphatides and lipoproteins. The blood of a healthy person always contains sufficient quantities of these essential ingredients, but without these, cancer cells grow wild and out of control.

Blood analysis of cancer patients showed a strange greenish-yellow substance in place of the healthy red oxygen carrying hemoglobin that belongs there. This discovery led Dr. Budwig to test her theory and she found that when these natural ingredients where consumed over approximately a three month period, tumors gradually receded. The strange greenish elements in the blood were replaced with healthy red blood cells as the phosphatides and lipoproteins reappeared. Weakness and anemia disappeared and life energy was restored. Symptoms of cancer, liver dysfunction and diabetes were alleviated.

Dr. Budwig's formula is reportedly used in Europe for prevention and treatment of many diseases, including cancer, arteriosclerosis, stroke, heart attack, irregular heartbeat, stomach ulcers, arthritis, eczema, and immune deficiency syndromes such as MS and autoimmune diseases such as lupus.

Omega 3 fatty acids (flaxseed oil)

The body requires special fats that, among other important functions, make it possible for sufficient oxygen to reach the cells via the cellular membranes. Despite all the concern about fat in our diet, the body does require healthy fats and oils to function. Researchers are studying the effects omega-3 fatty acids have on delaying or reducing tumor development in **breast and prostate cancer**. Called essential fatty acids, or EFAs, these special fats must be supplied from outside the body every day, from foods and certain oils, because our bodies can't manufacture them. The omega-3 fatty acids include alpha-linolenic acid, eicosapentaenoic acid and docosahexaenoic acid. Sources and recommended servings of foods naturally high in omega-3 fatty acids include **flaxseed oil** and beans such as kidney, great northern, navy, and soybeans.

Experiments have shown that the prime cause of cancer is too little oxygen getting into the cell. Think of these polyunsaturated EFAs as "oxygen magnets". After three decades of research Dr. Budwig discovered a totally natural formula that not only protects against the development of cancer, but helps reverse cancer illness. People all over the world who have been diagnosed with incurable cancer and sent home to die, have reportedly had remission and now lead normal healthy lives.

If taking pharmaceutical drugs, consult with your health care practitioner about using these highly essential nutrients.

Budwig claims that the absence of linol-acids [in the average western diet] is responsible for the production of oxydase, which induces cancer growth and is the cause of many other chronic disorders. The human body cannot function properly without two polyunsaturated fats - linoleic and alpha-linoleic acid, both of which are found in flaxseed oil. Recent research suggests that ALA (alpha-linoleic acid) and lignans in flaxseed modulate the immune response and may play a beneficial role in the clinical management of autoimmune diseases. Flax has been grown since the beginnings of civilization. Of all plant oils, flax oil is the richest source of these omega 3 acids (naturally occurring variations not considered).

Dr. Budwig discovered that these two natural foods, organic flax seed oil and cottage cheese, must be eaten together to be effective since one triggers the release of the properties of the other. When this oil is combined with protein in the form of sulphurated amino acids found in cottage cheese or quark (a dairy product readily available in German-speaking countries made from various types of milk and roughly similar to cottage cheese) it allows the highly unsaturated fatty acids to become water-soluble, thus bypassing the need for an often diseased or impaired liver to break down the unsaturated fat by its own efforts. This combination helps balance an oversupply of omega 6 fatty acids and hydrogenated fats in the Western diet and to provide an immediately available abundant supply of essential omega 3 acids.

When you mix together cottage cheese and flax seed (linseed oil) the fat becomes water-soluble" and thereby immediately available for use by the body, providing the necessary "spark plugs" for cells to "breathe", detoxify and function. This effect is even more pronounced when combining the flax oil cottage cheese mix with a sugar-free diet containing much raw organic food.

Dr. Budwig's diet (which, when properly applied, involves not only ingestion of the above oil-protein mixture, but also a healthy minimally processed vegetarian diet, freshly ground flaxseeds, sunlight, stress management, etc.) has literally pulled people back from death's doorstep. Based on this evidence and its ease of implementation, it may be the quickest and easiest move to take for many stricken with a cancer challenge and/or those who are looking for an often fast-working approach to health recovery.

Enzymes are important. Dr. Budwig had her patients
take papaya juice for enzymes. (Many people take
enzyme supplements).

Eat whole and natural foods - organic where possible.
Prepare foods fresh. Don't keep foods for the next meal
or the next day.

It is very important to avoid unwholesome foods and
substances such as hydrogenated fats, animal fats,
sugar, white flour, preservatives, chemicals and
processed foods.

3. **Essiac tea**

Originally developed by a nurse in Canada, Rene Caisse (Essiac is Caisse spelled backward) this is one of the oldest of all alternative cancer treatments. It is highly regarded by many alternative physicians.

Composed of Burdock, Indian Rhubarb, Sorrel, Slippery Elm and sometimes other ingredients, more recently some companies are substituting yellow dock herb or curly dock herb for the sheep sorrel. However, the original recipe stipulated **sheep sorrel**.

One thing to consider is that Rene Caisse made her own tea fresh when treating patients and it was administered to them within 48 hours of making it, whereas current Essiac Tea products have been dehydrated, processed and stored for maybe several months.

Nurse Caisse claimed the formula was given to her by Canadian Ojibway Indians and she had tremendous success with it, working with it for decades. She was arrested and jailed many times for "practicing medicine without a license" but hundreds of former cancer patients credited her for saving their lives.

There are some exceptions where people should NOT take Essiac Tea, particularly pregnant women and those with brain tumors, because the tea seems to initially make the tumor grow, before breaking down.

Essiac Tea it is considered to be a Stage 3 cancer treatment, suggesting it's not strong enough for Stage 4 treatment, although it might be effective for Stage 4 when used in combination with other treatments. Many alternative physicians use Essiac to help cleanse the blood, especially if a patient has been on chemotherapy or radiation.

4. **Wheat Grass – Wigmore Therapy:**

Wheatgrass juice has been proven over many years to benefit people in numerous ways: cleansing the lymph system, building the blood, restoring balance in the body, removing toxic metals from the cells, nourishing the liver and kidneys and restoring vitality. Anne Wigmore (1909-1993) originally devised the Wheatgrass juice and sprouts regimen to cure her own cancer and, for decades thereafter, she was successful in helping others using the same approach.

Wheat grass therapy consists of detoxification and consuming a wheat-grass drink several times each day. Fresh wheat grass in this form is a great source of many vitamins, minerals and plant enzymes and is said to be natures own nutritional program. It is a concentrated food and one ounce of wheatgrass juice has the vitamin and mineral equivalent of 2.2 pounds of fresh vegetables. It contains most of the vitamins and minerals needed for human maintenance, including B12. It also contains Amygdalin/Laetrile, although other sources, such as apricot seeds are more concentrated.

Wheatgrass juice is a living food, which is a complete protein with about 30 enzymes and is approximately

70% chlorophyll. In addition to wheat grass juice and sprouts, the Wigmore diet focuses primarily on live foods because she felt that raw vegetables held more nutrition than when cooked and were without the chemical additives that processed foods hold (organic grown foods are obviously best).

Growing your own wheat grass is preferable and you'll need a hand juicer for best results. Alternatively there are commercial juices available, but then price factor and freshness need to be considered. Another alternative is buying the wheatgrass in powdered form for mixing with water or other juices, such as red **grape juice**.

5. **Grapes and Red Wine:**

In the 1920s, Johanna Brandt of South Africa said she
cured her stomach cancer with what she called The
Grape Cure, which basically consists of consuming
nothing but **grapes** or **grape** juice. The diet routine is
very specific and readers who would like to know more
should do a search on "Johanna Brandt grape cure".

Purple grapes, complete with their skin and seeds and,
to a slightly lesser degree red and black grapes,
contain an amazing variety of antioxidants and several
nutrients that are known to kill cancer cells and help
stop the spread of cancer, plus detoxify the body.
Although many of these substances were unknown at
the time Brandt used this method, recent scientific
research confirms that many of these substances are
natural cancer killers.

However, some researchers warn against using this
diet solely, particularly with fast spreading cancers.
Some say it doesn't work for all cancers.

It's interesting to note that doctors a hundred years ago
in northern Europe were combining the "grape cure"
with other alternative practices. Other researchers have
found that Red grape skins contain a substance called

resveratrol, a naturally occurring phenol that inhibits cancer growth.

Red wine, even without alcohol, not only has resveratrol, found in grape skins, but also polyphenols that may protect against various types of cancer. Polyphenols are potent antioxidants, compounds that help neutralize disease-causing free radicals. Bearing in mind that alcohol can be toxic to the liver and to the nervous system, and that many wines have sulfites, which may be harmful to your health, it would be best to stick with grape juice. Some research indicates that alcohol is considered a class "A" carcinogen which can actually cause cancer.

6. **Food Grade Hydrogen Peroxide**

Food grade hydrogen peroxide (H2O2) is being touted by some to be the answer to many diseases. However, there are specific instructions and precautions around this method and you can have adverse reactions if you don't follow the guidelines. Have a look at the following site that gives a good overview of the pros and cons of this method:

http://www.cancertutor.com/hydrogenperoxide/

see also the related article
http://www.cancertutor.com/water_trick/

Some essential precautions include:

- Always use <u>Food Grade</u> hydrogen peroxide (not the product you get from your local drug store or health store that has additives and is intended for external use only).

- Preferably use 3% H2O2 – the 35% H2O2 is highly corrosive and can be dangerous to handle.

- Always dilute in distilled water (not tap water because minerals in water can react with the H2O2).

- When taking internally, always dilute with at least 4oz of distilled water (even when taking the 3% H2O2) and preferably use a glass container, not plastic.

- Do not take any other foods or drinks for at least 3 hours prior to taking H2O2 (nor for one hour after) because some foods react badly. In particular, don't take H2O2 within several hours of taking any anti-oxidants.

- Always start with low dose H2O2 - a couple of drops in distilled water three times a day and slowly build up to higher concentrations over a number of days as your body allows – never increase if you experience adverse stomach reactions.

Now, before you read on, make sure that you've taken in that it's food grade hydrogen peroxide, not the product that's available at you local drugstore, which has preservatives in it and is for external use only. There are several places online where you can buy food grade hydrogen peroxide, but there's a specific protocol for taking the substance and it's essential that you follow the correct method.

On its own it can be corrosive and it needs to be in specific dilutions. An important part here is that it should be taken with distilled water, available from you local food market. If used with ordinary tap water, the chlorine and other minerals in the water are accentuated and can result in adverse reactions. Most people would find it hard to stomach.

For those of you who are unsure of what hydrogen peroxide is, its chemistry symbol is H_2O_2 (two parts hydrogen to two parts oxygen) whereas ordinary tap water is H_2O (one part oxygen). By diluting the food grade hydrogen peroxide in distilled water the body is flooded with extra oxygen that permeates the cells and helps fight disease. It's as simple as that.

But as I said, there is a specific protocol and generally you start with a couple of drops in distilled water three times a day and slowly build up to higher concentrations. There are several books on the market that are specifically dedicated to this form of treatment. However, it's just one of several natural treatments that can be used for cancer.

Hydrogen peroxide can also be absorbed through the skin by having a peroxide bath – add a cup of 35% food grade hydrogen peroxide (or 10 cups of 3%) to a bathtub of warm water and soak for 20 to 30 minutes as the hydrogen peroxide is absorbed through the skin.

Before trying the Hydrogen Peroxide method internally, please reread the first paragraph of this section.

7. **Vitamin C:**

High dosages of Vitamin C is considered to be your body's best friend, particularly in cases of cancer. Apparently Vitamin C is one of the few vitamins that human beings, along with a small handful of other mammals, cannot make within their own bodies, therefore supplementation is essential, particularly if food derived Vitamin C is insufficient. Its uses in the body seem endless.

It has been known for many years that cancer patients have depressed circulating, cellular, and tissue ascorbate (vitamin C) reserves. Ascorbate is involved in many aspects of a person's resistance to cancer.

The suggested dosage should be taken every six hours (four times a day), and once commenced should never be abruptly discontinued because of the rebound effect. Recommendations vary, one suggesting that the dose, depending on the individual, should be in the 10 to 30g a day range. However, there are many differing opinions among health practitioners, where some believe that excess vitamin C is simply passed out of the body via the urine, but others believe that too high a dose puts strain on the liver.

One common agreement is the need for this vitamin, although the dose might vary between individuals. Check with your health professional.

8. **Apricot pits**

Thousands of people worldwide have made use of a key ingredient in apricot pits, a form of organic cyanide, to fight cancer. Amygdalin or vitamin B17 (also called Laetrile) is a powerful cancer fighter. There are various forms, including intravenous and pill forms of Laetrile available today, but this therapy still remains discredited and banned by the American government after many years of continuous use in other countries around the world.

Some people simply choose to eat apricot seeds, a rich natural source of Amygdalin, but remember … everything in moderation. Take note that nature provides one pit per fruit – eating too many pits at one time without the whole fruit is unbalanced and can cause an oversupply of Amygdalin, possibly toxic. The official position of the FDA is that doing this is contrary to their rulings and therefore subject to prosecution (apparently they do prosecute people for selling apricot pits). Some believe the seeds, which are contained within the pits, are superior to extracts as they contain other naturally occurring factors.

The value of the active ingredient, called nitrilosides (Amygdalin or Laetrile) has been discredited by the government and major drug manufacturers. Yet many people have pointed to this therapy as being responsible for finally eliminating their cancers.

Nitrilosides are also contained in over 1200 common fruits, nuts, grains and grasses. The trace of organic cyanide can effectively destroy cancer cells in early stages of the disease.

This therapy is usually used in conjunction with the proteolytic enzymes (see below), a broad-spectrum nutritional program and a diet consisting of fresh fruits and vegetables, whole grains, with no meat or dairy products for the duration of treatment.

Proteolytic enzymes (or proteases) refer to the various enzymes that digest (break down into smaller units) protein. These enzymes include the pancreatic proteases chymotrypsin and trypsin, bromelain (pineapple enzyme), papain (papaya enzyme) and fungal proteases.

Enzymes are proteins that facilitate chemical reactions in living organisms. They are required for every single chemical action that takes place in your body. All of your tissues, muscles, bones, organs and cells are run by enzymes. The vast majority of metabolic enzymes in the body – the enzymes that regulate everything from liver function to the immune system – are proteases, or proteolytic enzymes, which regulate protein function in the body. When we eat foods that are enzyme dead (cooked or processed), we force the body to divert its production of enzymes away from proteolytic enzymes, which govern metabolic functions, into enzymes designed to break down dead proteins in our diets.

This emphasizes the importance of a diet of fresh fruits and vegetables and supplementing with digestive proteolytic enzymes.

9. **Garlic:**

One of the best cancer fighting foods, garlic is
particularly good for Lung cancer, studies have shown
that garlic eaters have a striking risk reduction in oral,
esophageal, laryngeal, colorectal, breast, ovarian, and
prostate cancers. Studies have shown Garlic eaters
may cut their risk of stomach cancer in half, and their
risk of colon cancer by one-third. Risk reduction for
most cancers is an amazing 55 to 80 percent!

Hippocrates prescribed **garlic** as one of the best
cancer fighting foods and for many other conditions,
including parasites, poor digestion, respiratory
problems, and fatigue. This strong food has been
around for thousands of years. It was administered to
Olympic athletes in Greece and in ancient India they
not only revered it for its therapeutic properties, but
they believed it was an aphrodisiac as well.

Use fresh, chopped, or squeezed to get maximum
therapeutic benefit. Cooking reduces its enzymatic
action and garlic supplements are not as good as raw.
The secret of claiming garlic's anti-cancer benefits is to
Eat it raw – and crush it before eating!

However, a word of caution – although Garlic is one of the best cancer fighting foods, it can cause stomach upset, so start slowly and eat it with other foods.

Garlic is a natural blood thinner known for preventing plaque buildup linked to heart disease, stroke, and blood clots. Don't use a lot of garlic if you're on a blood thinner or on medications – check with your doctor.

Many people have trouble eating garlic straight up. It has the potential to cause distress, especially if taken raw on an **empty** stomach. Some ways of combining raw garlic with other foods can include homemade salsa (with fresh or canned tomatoes, onions and olive oil), Guacamole (garlic mixed with avocado), salad dressing (mixed with balsamic vinegar and herbs, particularly oregano and basil). You can also stir the crushed and diced garlic into your cooked vegetables and also mashed potatoes before serving, or ferment the garlic in salt brine.

If you want to avoid your breath and possibly your sweat from stinking, the best known cure is to eat fresh parsley with the garlic. That's why many garlic recipes, including garlic butter, include the green herb. Another option to avoid garlic breath is to chew on a cardamom pod after the meal – it sweetens the breath.

When preparing garlic, rubbing a little olive oil on the fingers helps prevent the garlic smell staying on the skin.

If you cook garlic, chop it and wait 10 minutes before cooking, allowing the enzymes to work and to try and maintain most of its benefits.

10. **Ginger:**

Ginger can be included in the list of natural cancer cures. Particularly good for **breast cancer** and **ovarian cancer**, an American study also showed that ginger extract helped kill **prostate cancer** cells *while letting healthy prostate cells live*. Ginger may also help fight other cancers such as colon, liver, lung, pancreas and skin cancers, including melanoma.

The researchers used ginger powder similar to that in your spice cabinet, but upgraded to a standardized research grade. Ginger showed the highly prized anti-cancer quality of selective cytotoxicity - it kills cancer cells but leaves healthy cells unharmed – one of the natural cancer cures.

The study used a daily dose of 100 mg of ginger extract per kg of body weight (about 6800 mg per day for a 150 pound person). If using fresh ginger, the researchers estimate 100 grams would offer similar results. With those quantities, if taking ginger to fight a pre-existing condition, then maybe an extract would be more tolerable. However, adding ginger to your daily diet is worth considering as one of the natural cancer cures for general wellbeing.

Researchers who've studied the healing properties of ginger discovered it contains zingibain, an enzyme with exceptionally strong anti-inflammatory properties. This might help explain how ginger fights cancer cells, as well as providing relief for arthritis sufferers and many other inflammation-mediated diseases.

Besides being one of the natural cancer cures, Ginger is thought to help fight diverticulitis, gallbladder inflammation, and heart disease - also to promote blood flow to your brain to keep it healthy and young. Used as a pain relief, it has no known side effects. Osteoarthritis and fibromyalgia are just two conditions that could benefit from ginger's pain relief. It is also believed to be good for the heart, stopping life-threatening platelet aggregation, hardening of the arteries, and high cholesterol.

However, a word of caution – ginger can have effects on some prescription drugs, so consult your doctor if you're on any, particularly heart or blood thinning meds or if you have a bleeding disorder. Ginger should never be given to children under two.

In China, ginger has been used to aid digestion and treat stomach upset, diarrhea, and nausea for over 2,000 years. A number of clinical trials show ginger, in addition to being one of the natural cancer cures, helps reduce the nausea and vomiting associated with chemotherapy It may also help people who suffer from Irritable Bowel Disease or IBS.

11. **Lemons for Fighting Cancer**

Lemon (Citrus) is a miraculous food for killing cancer cells, but it needs the whole lemon, particularly the skin. Simply place the washed lemon in the freezer section of your refrigerator and once the lemon is frozen, grate the whole lemon and sprinkle it on top of your foods.

Sprinkle it on your vegetable salad, ice cream, soup, cereals, noodles, spaghetti sauce, rice, sushi, etc. It enhances the taste of your food and you get the cancer fighting benefits! That's the lemon secret!

Lemon peels contain as much as five to ten times more vitamins than the lemon juice itself. By following this simple procedure of freezing the whole lemon, then grating it on top of your dishes, you can consume all of those nutrients and get even healthier. Lemon peels also help eradicate toxins in the body.

Lemons are a remedy against cancers of all types. They are also considered antimicrobial against bacterial infections and fungi, effective against internal parasites and worms. Lemons help regulate high blood pressure and are considered an antidepressant, combating stress and nervous disorders.

Lemon extract apparently destroys malignant cells in many cancers, including colon, breast, prostate, lung and pancreas. The compounds of this fruit slow the growth of cancer cells. And what is even more astonishing, therapy with lemon extract appears to only destroy malignant cancer cells without affecting healthy cells.

12. Coconut Oil Pulling

This is an unusual one and maybe a little controversial. Although it's not a specific cancer treatment as such, it aids in the general detoxification of the body and is beneficial in treating many illnesses.

 The term *Oil Pulling* refers to the drawing effect the oil has in pulling toxins out of the body via the tongue and mouth. It has its origins in Ayurvedic medicine, which dates back thousands of years, where *oil gargling* was practiced. However, the system used nowadays involves placing a vegetable oil in the mouth and swishing it around like a mouthwash, leaving it in the mouth for fifteen to twenty minutes before spitting it out. Although any vegetable oil can be used, organic coconut oil is recommended for its cleansing properties and fresh taste.

Sounds strange, but there are many reports of great results, not only in general oral hygiene, where even problems such as bleeding gums, tooth decay and gum disease are greatly diminished or healed, but it also has a powerful cleansing and healing affect on the entire body. Relief from illnesses such as asthma, allergies, chronic fatigue, diabetes, migraine headaches, PMS and chronic skin problems have been reported.

Oil pulling works by detoxifying or cleansing the body. Our mouths are the home to billions of bacteria, viruses, fungi and other parasites and toxins. By removing the disease promoting toxins, it allows the body to heal itself. From that perspective, this simple and low cost practice would be beneficial when adopting any natural healing protocol. It's best done first thing in the morning on an empty stomach. For more details, do an internet search on *Coconut Oil Pulling*.

Dietary Aids

1. Arginine (1-arginine)

Arginine is a vitally important amino acid that has been studied for more than fifty years. Amino acids are the building blocks of protein and protein is the building block of all living cells. Arginine has been found to consistently inhibit the growth of tumors.

There are several vegetable sources of dietary arginine – it is found in chocolate, wheat germ and flour, buckwheat, granola, oatmeal, dairy products (**cottage cheese**, ricotta, nonfat dry milk, skim yogurt), nuts (coconut, pecans, cashews, walnuts, **almonds**, Brazil nuts, hazel nuts, peanuts, seeds (pumpkin, sesame, sunflower), chick peas and cooked soybeans.

Arginine has been linked to enhanced immunity, the release of the Human Growth Hormone (HGH), greater muscle mass, rapid healing from injury, increased sexual potency and helping to reverse atherosclerosis. It increases the size and activity of the thymus gland, which is responsible for manufacturing T lymphocytes – the much talked about T-cells, which assist the immune system. It is also important in liver health and assists in neutralizing ammonia in the liver.

In 1980, National Cancer Institute scientists found that injections of arginine into tumor-bearing rats consistently inhibited the growth of tumors. Their reports stated, "within two weeks, tumor size was reduced to 80 percent of the initial size. Tumor-bearing animals showed no toxic effects from the arginine."

2. **Minimize Phosphorous in the diet**

This one comes from an Australian farmer who believes we have an oversupply of phosphorus in the food chain due to the use of superphosphates on crops and pasture land. In his book, *Cancer: Cause & Cure*, Percy Weston describes how, over many years, he saw the debilitating effects of phosphorus on livestock and humans. From observations and experiments over many years, it seems that phosphorus in the body could be a strong contributing factor in cancer cases.

Due to the widespread use of superphosphates, even dairy products and meat has high phosphorus content, including grain fed stock where the feed comes from superphosphate-dosed fields. Therefore, it's best to avoid meat and dairy, and consume organic produce where possible.

For many people, the cost or availability of organic produce is a big factor. Percy experimented and came up with a mix of salts that balance and absorb the phosphorus. The initial mix is noted below and he developed that further over time, adding additional salts in various quantities to produce a product that has had great results (do an internet search on *Percy Weston CAA* for details of where to buy the product).

The initial simple mix is an old household remedy and had good results. He identified magnesium as an essential element to balance phosphorus, so he made a mix of Epsom salts (sulphate of magnesium sulfur and oxygen) and Bicarbonate of soda (sodium and sulphates of potassium and iron). The mix (1 part Epsom salts to 4 parts Baking Soda) was designed to counter or neutralize phosphorus in the body and had the added advantage of relieving arthritis. He started with a quarter spoonful daily, taken in water and lemon juice, working up to a level spoonful. The principle is that ions of phosphorus (non-metal) combine with alkali (metallic) ions of potassium, magnesium etc. in solution and pass out through the urine.

3. **Tomatoes:**

Researchers have found that a diet rich in tomatoes might be a simple way to minimize the risk of illnesses such as cancer and heart disease, regardless of whether the tomatoes are eaten raw or cooked. Studies in various countries have found the same results, where a diet rich in tomatoes or tomato products, even tomato sauce, reduces the risk of cancer, with results ranging from 35 to 50%. The studies covered a variety of cancers, including prostate cancer, breast cancer, multiple myeloma (bone-marrow cancer) and renal cell carcinoma (a type of kidney cancer).

Scientists suspect that lycopene, a potent antioxidant found in the fruit, is responsible for the anti-cancer effect, although lycopene on its own is not as effective as the whole fruit, suggesting there are other properties in the whole food that compliment each other. Another benefit of eating tomatoes is that they appear to offer natural protection against skin damage from the sun.

One review showed that lycopene not only reduced the risk of prostate cancer, but might also delay prostate cancer progression, and reduce symptoms such as pain and urinary tract problems. Results also suggest that lycopene could be a complementary therapy for high-grade tumours (gliomas) of the brain or spine.

Further studies showed that Tomatoes may also help to prevent heart disease. The experiments showed that those who ate the most tomato-based products had a 30-per-cent lower risk of heart disease and a 60-per-cent reduced risk of heart attack. Short-term treatment with lycopene-rich tomato extract was found to reduce blood pressure in patients with hypertension.

4. **Kombu (seaweed delicacy) – Fucoidan**

Edible brown seaweeds have been a mainstay in Japanese cuisine for centuries. Regardless of the type, bladder wrack, kombu or wakame, which are all used in soups and other dishes in Japan, it's the compound fucoidan in the seaweed that is attracting the most interest due to its cancer fighting benefits.

Seaweed has also been used in Oriental medicine throughout history, the various types used for different purposes. Bladder wrack is a rich source of iodine, used to treat swelling of the thyroid gland (goiter), whereas Wakame has been used to purify the blood, promote intestinal function and improve skin and hair. But it's only since the 1970's that research into fucoidan started. These scientific studies confirmed that fucoidan causes certain types of rapidly growing cancer cells to die.

Fucoidan is a type of carbohydrate called a *polysaccharide* that's found in the cell walls of brown seaweed. It has a high nutritional value, rich in calcium, iodine, zinc, iron, selenium and vitamin A. These nutrients are essential for circulatory, immune and the neurologic systems function.

Ongoing clinical research shows fucoidan may prove to be a superstar cancer warrior. It induces *apoptosis*, or natural cell death, in cancer cells. Getting cancer cells to undergo apoptosis is one of the Holy Grails of cancer therapy. Fucoidan appears to trigger the mechanism that causes cancer cells to commit this biological suicide.

Packets of dried seaweed are available at your local oriental supply store. You can add a small serving to a little water and, within a few minutes, eat it raw as a snack or add a little miso paste and have it as a nutritious soup.

5. **Asparagus**

Alternative health experts rate glutathione as one of the most valuable antioxidants. Tests on asparagus show it is highest in glutathione (GSH), a phyto-chemical that's an antioxidant with cancer-fighting properties. Asparagus is also rich in cancer-blocking vitamins A (as beta-carotene) and C, as well as selenium, all fierce cancer fighters, plus anti-inflammatory properties and other vitamins like vitamin E, zinc and manganese, plus others.

It's the glutathione, a very special peptide molecule that's been dubbed the "Master Antioxidant" because it recharges other antioxidants and keeps them doing their job better and longer. GSH protects your genes from attack, disarms free radicals before they can wreak havoc and can help clean up already-existing damage. Studies show that glutathione strengthens your T cells, which help modulate your immune system and attack pathogens, while protecting your tissues and controlling autoimmune responses. It guards against cellular toxins and helps eliminate carcinogens.

Our body makes its own glutathione, but less every year as we age. When glutathione is deficient, toxins overload the liver and are stored in fat tissue, most often in the central nervous system, breasts, and prostate. Therefore, it's essential to boost the glutathione levels from food, and asparagus has the highest levels. It's best to get the glutathione in the whole food rather than in supplement form because it absorbs better into the body when taken with its other naturally occurring nutrients and precursors.

The anti-inflammatory nutrients in asparagus are excellent to help prevent inflammatory-related diseases like cancer. Since asparagus contains so many nutrients, it deserves a regular place in a healthy diet, along with other fruits and veggies. As a cancer treatment, a popular one with reportedly good results suggests using the full-stalk canned style asparagus, puree it and take 4 tablespoons in the morning and 4 tablespoons later in the day.

6. **Aloe**

With around three hundred variations of Aloe plants, it seems all have medicinal uses, but some are credited with far higher healing properties than others. Famous people throughout history have prized Aloe plants, including Hippocrates, the father of modern medicine, King Solomon, Alexander the Great and his teacher Aristotle. In the latter case it was the rare plant called *Aloe succotrina.*

Aloe contains life's basic building blocks, essential vitamins and minerals, proteins, polysaccharides, enzymes, and amino acids. The leaves are filled with gel, mainly water plus known nutrients, including twenty minerals, twelve vitamins, eighteen amino acids, two hundred active plant compounds such as phytonutrients, enzymes, proteins, oils, monosaccharides and polysaccharides.

Although most people use Aloe as a topical skin cream, the yellow bitter part of the leaf is a proven laxative and the whole-leaf extracts can boost the immune system, reduce swelling, improve healing, kill bacteria and viruses, and improve communication within and between cells. The effects are dependant on people's biochemistry, but generally it is credited to stopping the growth of tumor cells, lowering cholesterol / triglycerides, oxygenating the blood, easing inflammation, easing joint pain and alkalizing the body, balancing acid levels. There are many more benefits, particularly attributed to aloe arborescens, rather than the less potent and commonly known aloe vera.

The aloe arborescens protocol for cancer was developed by Father Romano Zago, a Catholic priest from Brazil, who wrote the book *Cancer Can Be Cured!* His experiments and results were specifically for aloe arborescens and the protocol consists of aloe with honey and a distillate, which can be combined with other alternative cancer treatments. See the final chapter in this publication for further details.

7. **Avocados**

A diet of healthy fruits and vegetables helps prevent cancer, but the avocado in particular shows tremendous potential for preventing certain types of cancer. Studies conducted by Ohio University showed that the nutritional value and high phytonutrient and phytochemical content of the Hass avocado helps thwart cancer cells. Avocados' nutrients not only kill cancer cells, but also prevent the development of pre-cancerous ones. It was particularly beneficial with oral cancer.

The proteins in avocados are easily digested, they provide an entire day's supply of omega-3 fatty acids, the good fat your body needs and what's sorely lacking in the Western diet. Although high in fat, sixty percent of it is monounsaturated and avocados contain no cholesterol. They also offer an array of carotenoids, including beta-carotene, alpha-carotene, and lutein, as well as lesser known types, enhancing immune and reproductive health.

Studies show that oleic acid, the primary fatty acid in avocados, improves cardiovascular health. Avocados are bursting with enzymes, are rich in minerals, including magnesium, B vitamins, as well as vitamins

A, C, E, and K. They contain more protein, beta carotene, potassium, magnesium, folic acid, thiamin, riboflavin, niacin, biotin, pantothenic acid, vitamin E and vitamin K per ounce than any other fruit.

In particular, avocados contain 17.7 mg of glutathione per 100 g of raw edible fruit, more than three times that of any other fruit. Studies link high glutathione intake with a lowered risk of oral cancer and pharyngeal cancer, and quite likely other cancers also.

The reduced risk of cancer only occurred with the glutathione from raw fruits and veggies, so this is another case for including higher amounts of raw food in your diet, especially avocados.

8. **Berries – particularly Black Raspberries**

While strawberries, red raspberries, blackberries, and blueberries are generally regarded as cancer-fighting and healthy, studies show **black raspberries** may be even more powerful, especially against colon cancer and esophageal cancer. The black raspberry's darker skin means it contains significantly higher levels of cancer-fighting anthocyanins than do red raspberries, plus many other cancer-fighting phytochemicals, vitamins, minerals, and acids.

Besides a high antioxidant value, the black raspberry has anti-inflammatory and neuro-protective benefits, which might be particularly helpful in preventing colorectal cancer and esophageal cancer. In an experiment where mice were engineered to get tumors, the ones randomly fed black raspberry powder had the number of new tumors slashed by forty-five percent, and the number of total tumors by sixty percent. Research suggests that the black raspberry's ability to fight inflammation in the body may be linked to its ability to fight cancer, and perhaps also other diseases of aging as well.

Black raspberries and blackberries look similar, so if you're picking and eating the fruit fresh, the way to tell the difference is, raspberries leave a little white core behind when you pull the fruit off the bush, whereas blackberry cores come off with the fruit. The black raspberry is more seedy and less juicy.

Black raspberries aren't found often in stores, so a convenient way to take the required amount of about two cups a day is to buy the freeze dried powder form or take a black raspberry supplement. Both options are available via the internet if not from your local store and both options allow you to take more concentrated amounts, although supplements will generally contain less fructose than the powder, and therefore fewer calories.

All the most common and popular berries, strawberries, blueberries and blackberries as well as raspberries, have tremendous health benefits, so it's advisable to include them regularly in your daily diet. Buy organic because large amounts of chemicals are used in growing berries the conventional way.

9. **Papaya**

Research on foods that had ability to stop breast cancer cell growth found that papaya was high up there compared with other foods. The key ingredient might be organo-sulfer compounds called isothiocyanates, which experiments have found to be effective against cancers of the breast, lung, pancreas, colon and prostate, also leukemia.

10. Ginseng

Asian healers have used ginseng root for thousands of years to treat digestive and respiratory ailments, nervous disorders, diabetes and fatigue. In recent years Western scientists have been studying ginseng for its potential medicinal benefits, including possible anticancer properties. Most of the research has focused on three types of ginseng, although botanists have identified 12 species of ginseng.

The three ginseng types used in the study were **Panax ginseng** (Korean ginseng) , **Panax quinquefolium** (American ginseng) and **Panax notoginseng** — cultivated in Yunnan and Guangxi provinces in China. Of these three, the first two are the most commonly available in the West, either as extract or powdered root.

The studies revealed that compounds called ginsenosides are the plant's key ingredient for fighting cancer and the scientists identified four ways ginsenosides may shut down cancer cells:

I. **Arrest uncontrolled growth** - ginsenosides have been shown to halt growth of tumor cells in the liver, lungs and prostate, also leukuemia cells.

II. **Cause cell death** - substances found in ginsenosides apparently cause apoptosis (normal self-destruction) of lung, ovarian and prostate cancer cells, and also in nerve tissue (neuroblastoma).

III. **Halt invasive spreading** - scientists observed that ginsenosides stopped the invasiveness of some endometrial cancer cells.

IV. **Stunt growth of new blood vessels** - the growth of new blood vessels from existing ones is called *angiogenesis* and is the way cancer feeds itself. A number of studies have shown that ginsenosides inhibited angiogenesis in different animal models.

As a general tonic, ginseng is used widely and is generally considered safe. When taken in higher doses, some people experience headaches, increased heart rate, nausea and restlessness or hyperactivity. As always, it's best to check with your health professional.

Combating Skin Cancer

Although the standard treatment for skin cancer is surgery, chemotherapy and radiation, there has also been an alternative 'Black Salve' topical treatment available for many years, though most people have never heard of it. The man who first spread the word about healing from black salve was Harry Hoxsey, founder of the "Hoxsey method".

Hoxsey is the great-grandson of John Hoxsey, an American physician who discovered a remarkable cancer treatment in 1840 after watching horses with cancer cure themselves by grazing on specific herbs they instinctually searched out. Harry Hoxsey had no formal medical training, but began promoting his great-grandfather's original cancer formula which contained the herbs, bloodroot, burdock, red clover, pokeroot, barberry root, buckthorn, prickly ash, stillingia root and cascara.

These days, there are many variations of the Black Salve herbal compound, but the base ingredient is bloodroot, chosen for its fast acting, powerful effect on a wide array of skin problems. It is a non-discriminating killer of abnormal cell clusters of almost any kind of abnormality. It is claimed that the alkaloids in bloodroot kill cancer cells, while leaving normal cells undamaged. The main thing to consider when buying a bloodroot paste is the fineness of the composition. The bloodroot has to be ground very fine to be effective, whereas courser variations are not as good. Best to search for review feedback to source the best product.

Sometimes the better black salve bloodroot paste is hard to find. An alternative treatment for skin cancer lesions is an extract from the common eggplant, as noted next.

Eggplant Treatment for Skin Cancer

There is a phytochemical in the common eggplant that is reported to be effective in treating skin cancer. It's not quite as simple as putting a slither of eggplant on the skin, but still quite easy to prepare. You can either buy the cream or tincture of the extract solasodine glycoside (BEC5), or you can make your own.

For the home variation simply dice a medium size eggplant (preferably organic) and place in a jar, then fill the jar with organic apple cider vinegar to cover the eggplant pieces. Put the mix in the refrigerator and leave for five to six days, giving the sealed jar a good shake once a day.

After six days the vinegar will have turned a darker shade – strain off the liquid to use this as the tincture. Store in a sealed jar and refrigerate.

To use the tincture on skin cancer areas, simply dip a cotton ball into the liquid and place on the lesion with a sticking plaster. Replace this daily until the area is healed.

Note: some have reported very good results using this simple method alone. Others have recommended adding a little Frankincense essential oil along with the eggplant tincture. Some prefer to alternate the treatments, using the Frankincense (diluted in a carrier oil like coconut or olive oil) directly on the lesion for a day, then using the eggplant tincture the next day.

Herbal Teas for Combating Cancer

Readers are encouraged to research the internet for additional information on these items.

Chamomile Tea
A super powerful chemical found in chamomile tea is reported to not only block   the spread of cancer, but shortens the life of existing cancer cells. The magic ingredient is called apigenin, a chemical that research has found to play a role in gene regulation. It seems to reprogram the cancer cells to act more like normal cells, dying off at their normal time. Chamomile is a daisy-like flower that, when dried, makes a pleasant tasting tea. It's commonly used in German and Hungarian herbal remedies.

Green Tea
Recent studies from Japan demonstrate that green tea, a popular cancer preventative and a favorite of the Asians for centuries, goes way beyond its role as a well-known antioxidant. If the study is confirmed, the secret lies in its telomerase inhibiting properties (one of the factors that sets cancer cells apart from normal cells is that they have telomerase, an enzyme that maintains telomeres on the ends of DNA). Japanese researchers have been able to show that green tea

extract (ECGC) inhibits telomerase of cancer cells in two different types of cancers in the test tube: leukemia and the solid tumor type. Researches have said "Green tea cannot prevent every cancer, but it's the cheapest and most reliable method for cancer prevention available to the general public." Extracts of green tea in pill form are now available.

Pau D'Arco

This South American herb is developing a reputation as an effective cancer fighter when taken daily as a tea over several months, but it must be brewed correctly and a maintenance dose must be consumed daily on an ongoing basis. Pau D'Arco has been used for many illnesses for centuries and is a favorite in all health food stores.

Red Clover

Often made into a tea, Red Clover apparently has 4 anti-tumor compounds. It is also a key ingredient in many cancer-treatment tea combinations, including Essiac tea, which is covered in more detail earlier on in this publication.

Herbs and Spices for Combating Cancer

Readers are encouraged to research the internet for additional information on these items.

Turmeric & Oregano

Spices and herbs have been used in cuisine since the beginning of time, but the health properties of these are often underestimated. From a healing perspective, two highly rated ones are Turmeric and Oregano. Other herbs and spices are covered later, but these two deserve special mention.

In traditional Indian Ayurvedic medicine, turmeric is considered one the most valuable cancer preventing foods. It has strong medicinal antioxidant, anti-inflammatory, immune enhancing and detoxifying properties, and it is believed that taking half a teaspoon of turmeric per day in the diet could eliminate DNA damage characteristic of aiding cancer development. Although traditionally used in cooking, especially curries, the turmeric can be taken in warm or hot water as a drink.

Besides its cancer fighting properties, turmeric has many other healing attributes. It's a blood purifier, helps cleanse the liver, aids digestion and suppresses inflammation in the stomach; prevents & treats ulcerations of all kinds including gastritis & colitis. Also good for skin problems and arthritis, taking half a teaspoon of turmeric daily in a little warm water is a good habit regardless of any health issues.

Oregano, the herb used more extensively in Western diets, is attracting attention for its cancer fighting properties, particularly prostate cancer. Earlier research showed that pizza seems to reduce cancer risk and it was initially thought that lycopene, which is found in the tomato sauce covering on pizzas, provided the main anti-cancer qualities. More recent research suggests that it's a combination of the lycopene with the oregano herb that creates a synergistic power punch. The research showed that carvacrol, a constituent of oregano, is causing apoptosis or cell death, particularly in prostate cancer cells.

This of course is no endorsement for living on pizza, but combining tomatoes and oregano in sauces for cooking would be beneficial.

Artemisinin

A Chinese herb, sweet wormwood (*qinghao* in Chinese). Specific breast cancer research apparently found that breast cancer cells treated with artemisinin and an iron-enhancing molecule (transferring) resulted

in an amazing decrease in breast cancer cells within 16
hours. The research pointed to the involvement of free
iron in the toxic effect of artemisinin toward cancer
cells, while basically sparing healthy cells.

Curcumin

Curcumin (diferuloyl methane) is the active compound
in the spice Tumeric and is claimed to be the reason for
the low incidence of breast cancer in India because of
the common use of the yellow spices in the local
cuisine. Even curry powder apparently helps stop the
spread of breast cancer because turmeric is a principal
ingredient in curry. Tumeric is a member of the ginger
family and is believed to have medicinal properties
because it inhibits production of the inflammation-
related enzyme cyclo-oxygenase 2 (COX-2), levels of
which are abnormally high in certain inflammatory
diseases and cancers. Researchers found that
curcumin inhibits the spread of breast cancer into the
lungs and improves the effectiveness of current
remedies. Curcumin is believed to directly induce
cancer cell apoptosis (cell suicide).

Cat's Claw

Uña de Gato,"cat's claw", is a thorny liana vine reputed
to be a remarkably powerful immune system booster

and effective in treating a wide array of maladies including cancer, systemic candidiasis, genital herpes, and AIDS. The highly effective properties contained in the inner bark of the cat's claw plant have demonstrated, through centuries of usage dating back to the time of the ancient Incas, to have a profound and positive influence on the body's defense system. Urarina tribesman of Peru tell stories of Una de Gato curing tumors.

Chinese Scullcap

Recent clinical studies indicate the herb Chinese skullcap from the mint family may deserve recognition as a cancer killer. Emphasis here is on Chinese Skullcap, not to be confused with American Skullcap. With Chinese Skullcap the root is used, whereas with the American herb the leaves are used.

In Chinese culture the plant known as Chinese skullcap (Sculletaria baicalensis) has been used throughout history for shrinking tumors, killing bacterial infections, reducing inflammation (also relevant to cancer), plus serving as a diuretic, treating hepatitis and more. Usually taken in extract or capsule (powdered) form, but when buying, do make sure it is derived from the **Chinese Skullcap**.

Graviola

Nearly 25 years ago it was discovered that the leaf of the Peruvian Graviola tree contained natural compounds having exceptional ability to prevent abnormal cellular division. Research has apparently shown that the tree's chemical extracts attack and destroy cancer cells with lethal precision. It is said t exhibit the ability to selectively hunt down and kill cancer cells without harming healthy cells and research has apparently shown it to effectively target and kill malignant cells in 12 different types of cancer, including colon, breast, prostate, lung, and pancreatic cancer. Today it is commonly available on the Internet in pill or liquid form.

Mistletoe

Although not recognized or accepted in many countries, doctors in Germany reportedly treat more than 50% of their cancer patients with mistletoe, with fantastic results. Mistletoe, a natural alternative cancer treatment, is a powerful medicinal plant used to treat many things, although it's especially deadly on cancer tumors.

It's often taken in extract form. An Australian study tested different varieties and found the extract called Fraxini, obtained from ash trees, was highly effective against colon cancer cells, while being less toxic to healthy cells than the other tested extracts. According to the Adelaide study Fraxini was more potent than chemotherapy. However, although it reduced the incidence of cancer cells when used by itself, it also improved chemo's potency against cancer cells when the two were used together.

Although considered a natural alternative cancer treatment, Mistletoe extract is also recognized by many doctors in Germany. A 2002 German study followed 10,000 people who suffered from colon, rectal, stomach, and breast cancers. Apparently the patients treated with mistletoe extract with brand name Iscador survived 40% longer, on average, than did patients in the control group.

Recent studies show it also helps in cases of ovarian and pancreatic cancer. According to some sources, an eight year study of 800 colon cancer patients found that patients treated with Iscador had fewer side effects, more relief from symptoms and were more likely to survive disease-free than patients in the control group.

Red Clover

Used for centuries, Red Clover can be used as a tea or in extract form and is believed to have at least four anti-tumor compounds.

Rosemary

Often used as a seasoning, it can also be consumed as a tea. An extract of rosemary, termed carnosol, has purportedly inhibited the development of both breast and skin tumors in animals and may help increase the activity of detoxification enzymes.

Saw Palmeto

Taken more commonly in extract form, Saw Palmeto is often used in the treatment of prostate cancer.

Specific Foods for Combating Cancer

Although all food varieties have their specific properties for combating various forms of cancer and other ailments, the following have shown specific properties that would be beneficial to include on a regular basis with a well balanced diet. Some are repeated due to their importance.

Kombu (seaweed delicacy) – Fucoidan

Kombu, a seaweed delicacy favored by the people in Okinawa, Japan, contains a long chain carbohydrate, called fucoidan, which scientists believe is why Okinawans rarely get any kind of cancer. Okinawa also has the world's highest percentage of people over 100. Fucoidan, sometimes referred to as U-fucoidan, appears to have an amazing array of health producing properties, including the fact that it is lethal to most types of cancer cells.

Garlic has immune-enhancing allium compounds (dialyl sultides) that appear to increase the activity of immune cells that fight cancer and indirectly help break down cancer causing substances. Studies have linked garlic - as well as onions, leeks, and chives - to lower risk of stomach and colon cancer.

Grapes, red contain bioflavonoids, powerful antioxidants that work as cancer preventives, and also ellagic acid, a compound that blocks enzymes that are necessary for cancer cells. Grapes are also a rich source of resveratrol, which inhibits the enzymes that can stimulate cancer-cell growth and suppress immune response.

Mushrooms - There are a number of mushrooms that appear to help the body fight cancer and build the immune system. They contain a protein called lectin, which attacks cancerous cells and prevents them from multiplying. One in particular is maitake, although that is only one of several mushroom types that are known for their cancer fighting properties. Some superfood mixtures, a blend of various mushrooms, are available for buying via the internet. Do your own internet search for those superfood options.

Nuts contain the antioxidants quercetin and campferol that may suppress the growth of cancers.

Almonds (not a nut, but a seed) are especially recommended for their cancer combating properties.

Brazil nut contains 80 micrograms of selenium, which is important for those with prostate cancer, but it is important to not overdo the dose – two per day is ample.

Walnuts are particularly recommended as a preventative for cancer. In experiments on mice that were genetically programmed to develop prostate cancer, a control group that were feed walnuts had a massive 60% reduction in cancer development.

(Note: Many people are allergic to the proteins in nuts, so if you have any symptoms such as itchy mouth, tight throat, wheezing, etc. after eating nuts, stop. Consider taking a selenium supplement instead or work with someone on how to eliminate this allergy.)

Tomatoes – covered in detail earlier in this publication and also listed in the next section.

Common Food properties for Combating Specific Cancers

Avocados are rich in glutathione, a powerful antioxidant that attacks free radicals in the body by blocking intestinal absorption of certain fats. Scientists also believe that avocados may also be useful in treating viral hepatitis (a cause of liver cancer), as well as other sources of liver damage.

Broccoli, cabbage, and cauliflower have a chemical component called indole-3-carbinol that can combat breast cancer. Broccoli sprouts have shown a consistent level of sulforaphane, which induces the production of certain enzymes that can deactivate free radicals and carcinogens, as much as 20 times higher than the levels found in mature heads of broccoli.

Carrots contain beta carotene, which may help reduce a wide range of cancers including lung, mouth, throat, stomach, intestine, bladder, prostate and breast. However, it is recommended not to cook the carrots.

Chili peppers and jalapenos contain a chemical, capsaicin, which may neutralize certain cancer-causing

substances (nitrosamines) and may help prevent
cancers such as stomach cancer.

Cruciferous vegetables - broccoli, cauliflower, kale,
Brussels sprouts, and cabbage contain two
antioxidants, *lutein and zeaxanthin* that may help
decrease prostate and other cancers.

Figs apparently have a derivative of benzaldehyde,
considered to be highly effective at shrinking tumors.
Fig juice is reportedly also a potent bacteria killer in
test-tube studies.

Grapefruits, like oranges and other citrus fruits,
contain monoterpenes, believed to help prevent cancer.
Some studies show that grapefruit may inhibit the
proliferation of breast-cancer cells in vitro.

Kale has isothiocyanates and phytochemicals, thought
to suppress tumor growth and block cancer-causing
substances from reaching their targets.

Licorice root has a chemical, glycyrrhizin, that blocks
a component of testosterone and therefore may help
prevent the growth of prostate cancer. But it comes

with a warning that excessive amounts can lead to elevated blood pressure, so everything in moderation.

Oranges and lemons contain limonene which stimulates cancer-killing immune cells.

Papayas have vitamin C folacin (also known as folic acid), which has been shown to minimize cervical dysplasia and certain cancers.

Raspberries contain many vitamins, minerals, plant compounds and antioxidants known as anthocyanins that may protect against cancer. Black raspberries are rich in antioxidants, thought to have even more cancer-preventing properties than blueberries and strawberries and may also thwart colon cancer.

Seaweed and other sea vegetables contain high concentrations of the minerals, plus beta-carotene, protein, vitamin B12, fiber, and chlorophyll, as well as chlorophylones - important fatty acids that may help in the fight against breast cancer.

Soy products like tofu contain several types of phytoestrogens — weak, nonsteroidal estrogens that could help prevent both breast and prostate cancer, although some people believe that high consumption of soy products could cause hormone imbalances that stimulate cancer growth.

Sweet potatoes contain many anticancer properties, including beta-carotene.

Tapioca is derived from the **cassava** plant. It is one of the many plants that manufactures cyanide (laetrile, B17).

Tomatoes contain lycopene, an antioxidant that attacks roaming oxygen molecules, known as free radicals, that are suspected of triggering cancer. It is concentrated by cooking tomatoes and recent studies indicate that for proper absorption, the body also needs some oil along with lycopene. Scientists in Israel have shown that lycopene can kill mouth cancer cells and an increased intake of lycopene has already been linked to a reduced risk of breast, prostate, pancreas and colorectal cancer.

Ultraviolet Light Therapy

This is one treatment that you won't be able to do at home, but something to consider with your medical professional.

This treatment goes back a long way, seventy years or more. It has the added advantage that it seems to have virtually no side effects other than good health. The treatment is relatively inexpensive and is reported to have had a good effect for many diseases, such as lupus, allergies, rheumatoid arthritis and many other illnesses including cancer.

You'll need a minimum of four treatments depending on the illness and, as mentioned above, you'll require help from your medical professional with this type of therapy. The good news is that there are a number of alternative doctors that can also provide this treatment.

It's relatively simple and was first discovered in 1928 by Emmitt Knott, a scientist who was experimenting with light when assisting the treatment of a woman who had a major infection. He took a sample of her blood and exposed it to ultraviolet light before reinfusion of the treated blood back into her arm. That simple treatment resulted in her body healing itself over time. It was taken seriously by the medical profession until the 1950's when antibiotics and vaccines took precedence as the main treatment for infections.

If you want to check out the ultraviolet light treatment option with your medical professional or alternative doctor, the treatment goes by many names, the most common of which is UBI or Ultraviolet Blood Irradiation. However it's also known as ultraviolet blood therapy or UVB, hematologic oxidative therapy, photo-luminescence, Biophotonic therapy, photo-oxidation therapy and a number of other names.

The basic treatment is fairly simple, using a butterfly needle and a syringe, where approximately 40-60 cubic centimeters (cc) of blood is taken from the arm. The blood is then mixed with a saline solution and that's an important part of the process because blood needs to be diluted for the ultraviolet light to be able to penetrate. It also makes the treatment easier to administer. With this dilution, of approximately 12% of blood and 88% saline, the absorption rate of the ultraviolet light is close to 100%. It only takes around thirty seconds of ultraviolet light to treat the blood solution before it is reintroduced back into the patient's arm. This treatment has also been known to treat shingles within only a couple of days.

It all sounds fairly simple – and it should be relatively inexpensive. However, treatment costs can vary, so it's advisable to shop around to find who is actually providing that service and at what cost. Of course, because your blood is being taken, treated and returned to your arm, it's important to get a professional who is experienced in this type of treatment.

As mentioned above, the UBI treatment is not a simple do it yourself option, but it's included here for those who would like to pursue this with their medical professional. If you do decide to go this way it would be better to include it as part of an overall health regime that combines a number of treatments as noted previously.

Be prepared for a skeptical response from medical doctors because there's not a lot of research confirming that this treatment works. However, it's an option well worth considering and there are a lot of people who have reported a positive result using this method.

The Power of Aloe

One simple plant that can be grown in your own back yard, or bought ready to go, has been used for thousands of years to promote health. The humble aloe plant detoxifies the body, renews the blood and strengthens the immune system.

Now before we go into more detail we need to mention there are several varieties of aloe, the most common one being Aloe Vera. However, the aloe we're talking about here is the one recommended by Father Romano Zago, a Brazilian priest who authored the book *Cancer Can Be Cured!* The aloe he recommends is Aloe Aroberscens.

This variety of aloe is not as common as the Aloe Vera, but can still easily be sourced with a simple internet search of your local area. You can either buy the plant and grow it yourself or purchase it ready to go if you prefer.

According to reports, Father Zago's treatment has had very positive results for various types of cancer. Skeptics might say that the main composition of aloe is water, but the plant also has staggering amounts of nutrients, enzymes, proteins, oils, amino acids, vitamins and minerals and active plant compounds. In short, the nutrients super charge your immune system, enabling your own body to fight cancer and other diseases.

In preparation of the leaves for use in this formula, you need to remove the spines from the leaves with a sharp knife, cut the leaves into pieces and put them into a blender with honey and distillate.

Here's Father Zago's formula:

- 0.77 lbs. of Aloe arborescens leaves (about 3-4 large leaves)
- 1.1 lbs. of honey (no synthetic or refined honey, only raw, pure pesticide-free honey)
- 2-3 tablespoons of distillate (grappa, whisky, cognac, or Mexican tequila — wine, beer, and liqueurs cannot be used)

Once blended, keep the solution in a dark container in the refrigerator.

As a treatment for cancer, he recommends taking a tablespoon of the mixture three times a day, one spoonful up to half an hour before each meal. Follow this regime for ten days and then stop for ten days, before resuming for another ten days. The treatment continues until the cancer disappears.

One thing to remember here is that the honey in the solution is heavier than the other ingredients, so will settle in the container. It's important to shake the mixture well before each use.

Father Zago emphasizes that all the ingredients are important, including the honey, which cleanses and removes impurities, and the alcohol, which helps dissolve the bitterness released by the aloe. It also helps dissolve the viscous composition of the aloe. He emphasizes that the formula contains aloin, which the body can't absorb unless it's dissolved in the alcohol. However, the proportion of the alcohol compared with the other ingredients is relatively low.

For those who want to try Aloe Vera instead of the Aloe Aroberscens, the Aloe Vera will still have a positive response, although it only contains 40% of the active ingredients needed to fight cancer, whereas the Aloe Aroberscens contains 70%. Therefore, if you can get the Aloe Aroberscens, it's the better choice.

For the most positive effect, also try and follow the recommended guidelines:

1. Preferably the Aloe plant should be five years old or more.
2. It's best not to pick the aloe within five days of rain because that just adds extra water in the mix.
3. It's best to pick, prepare and also drink the mixture in the dark because the aloe's cancer fighting substances are depleted by ultraviolet light and infrared rays.
4. It's best to prepare the mixture as soon as possible after picking the leaves to retain freshness.

Although the aloe treatment has relatively few side effects, the initial treatment may result in darkened urine, diarrhea or rashes. This occurs generally from the release of toxins from the body and is only a temporary thing.

For more details of the recipe and ready-made options, do a google search on *Father Zago's Brazilian formula* and particularly google search *The Plant that Cures Practically Everything.*

Bibliography and Recommended Sites:

Wisdom Wellness Diet – Returning to Health

Cancer: Cause & Cure: Percy Weston – BookBin Publishing Pty Ltd

Cancer Can Be Cured! Father Romano Zago – iUniverse publishing

http://cancertutor.com/

http://www.cancure.org/

http://www.cancerdefeated.com

Other Self Help Books by the Author

Wisdom Wellness Diet – Returning to Health

Self Sufficiency Survival - Easy to follow Guide and Manual

Other Fiction Books by the Author

Star Bred Prophecy ... A Time to Re-Member

The Blue Star Millennium – the original story (now Aaden BlueStar Awakening)

Quest for Genesis – A Journey of Discovery

Aaden BlueStar Awakening

Notes:

Notes:

Notes:

Notes:

Notes:

Notes:

Notes:

Notes:

www.ingramcontent.com/pod-product-compliance
Lightning Source LLC
Chambersburg PA
CBHW070718250726
48662CB00001B/480